THE PALEO DIET COOKBOOK FOR DIGESTIVE HEALTH

Restore Gut Balance And Improve Digestion With 100 Healthy Recipes

A 5 Days Meal Plan To Heal Your Gut And Alleviate Symptoms Of Digestive Disorders

Dr. Belinda Bianca

Table of Contents

CHAPTER ONE

Introduction

The Paleo Diet, also known as the Paleolithic or Caveman Diet, is a nutritional plan based on foods that are thought to have been accessible to humans during the Paleolithic period.

This diet focuses on whole foods including lean meats, fish, fruits, vegetables, nuts, and seeds, while avoiding processed foods, grains, dairy, and legumes. While the Paleo Diet is often used to lose weight and improve general health, its influence on digestive health is substantial and worth investigating.

Understanding The Paleo Diet:

The Paleo Diet focuses on eating foods that our predecessors would have hunted or collected. It stresses nutrient-dense natural foods above processed foods, grains, dairy, and legumes.

Proponents of the Paleo food say that by emulating our ancient ancestors' food, it is more aligned with our evolutionary biology, resulting in better health benefits.

10 Ways The Paleo Diet Improves Digestive Health:

Promotes Gut Microbiome Diversity:

The Paleo Diet, which is high in fruits, vegetables, and nuts, offers enough fiber and prebiotics to support healthy gut bacteria, resulting in a more diversified microbiome and greater digestive health.

Reduces Inflammation:

By avoiding processed foods and gluten-containing grains, the Paleo Diet helps to decrease inflammation in the gut, which alleviates symptoms of digestive illnesses such as Irritable Bowel Syndrome (IBS) and Crohn's.

Balances Blood Sugar Levels:

By emphasizing whole foods and eliminating processed sugars and grains, the Paleo Diet helps to regulate blood sugar levels, lowering the risk of insulin resistance and supporting improved digestive function.

Improves Nutrient Absorption:

Whole foods on the Paleo Diet are high in important nutrients and are more readily absorbed by the body than processed meals, promoting proper digestive function and nutrient absorption.

Eliminates Gut Irritants:

The Paleo Diet eliminates foods like grains, beans, and dairy, which contain substances that may irritate the gut lining and cause digestive pain. Removing these irritants may help with symptoms of leaky gut syndrome.

Enhances Digestive Enzyme creation:

The Paleo Diet's diversity of whole foods encourages the creation of digestive enzymes, which help in nutrient breakdown and absorption, hence enhancing overall digestive function.

Weight control:

The Paleo Diet's emphasis on full, nutrient-dense meals aids with appetite regulation and satiety, thus aiding in weight control and lowering the risk of obesity-related digestive diseases.

Reduces the Risk of Food Sensitivities:

By removing common allergens and irritants like gluten and dairy, the Paleo Diet may help detect and manage food sensitivities, resulting in better digestive comfort and general well-being.

Encourages Hydration:

Many Paleo-friendly meals, such as fruits and vegetables, are rich in water, which promotes hydration while also supporting healthy digestive function by reducing constipation and bowel regularity.

Provides Antioxidant Support:

The Paleo Diet's abundance of fruits and vegetables contains antioxidants that help counteract oxidative stress and inflammation in the digestive system, boosting overall gut health.

List Of 15 Common Digestive Disorders:

- Irritable Bowel Syndrome(IBS)
- Gastro esophageal reflux disorder (GERD)
- Crohn's disease.
- Ulcerative Colitis.
- Celiac disease.
- Diverticulitis
- Peptic Ulcers.

- Gallstones

- Hemorrhoids

- Constipation

- Diarrhea

- Gastritis

- Lactose intolerance

- Leaky Gut Syndrome.

- Small intestinal bacterial overgrowth (SIBO).

Foods To Include In The Paleo Diet For Digestive Health:

Lean Meats: Grass-fed beef, poultry, and wild-caught fish have high-quality protein and important nutrients with no additional hormones or antibiotics.

Fruits: Berries, apples, pears, and citrus fruits are high in fiber, vitamins, and antioxidants, which promote digestive health and regularity.

Vegetables: Leafy greens, cruciferous vegetables, and root vegetables include fiber, vitamins, and minerals that are necessary for proper digestive function.

Nuts and Seeds: Almonds, walnuts, chia seeds, and flaxseed are high in healthy fats, fiber, and minerals that promote gut health.

Healthy Fats: Avocado, coconut oil, and olive oil provide vital fatty acids that promote gut lining integrity and decrease inflammation.

Fermented foods such as sauerkraut, kimchi, and kombucha include probiotics, which support healthy gut microbiota and assist digestion.

Bone Broth: High in collagen and amino acids, bone broth promotes gut lining integrity and alleviates digestive pain.

Herbs and spices: Ginger, turmeric, and peppermint have anti-inflammatory and digestive characteristics that may help with stomach issues.

Coconut Products: Coconut milk, coconut flour, and shredded coconut are all gluten-free options high in fiber and healthy fats.

Pasture-raised eggs are high in protein, vitamins, and minerals, all of which promote digestive health.

Foods To Avoid On The Paleo Diet For Digestive Health:

Grains including wheat,   barley,   and rye contain gluten and other chemicals that may irritate the gut lining and worsen digestive problems.

Legumes: Beans, lentils, and peanuts include lectins and phytates, which may impair nutritional absorption and cause stomach discomfort.

Dairy products include lactose and casein, which may be difficult to digest for certain people and aggravate stomach problems.

Packaged snacks, sugary drinks, and processed meats often include chemicals and preservatives that might disturb gut bacteria and cause inflammation.

Refined Sugars: High-fructose corn syrup, cane sugar, and artificial sweeteners can disturb the gut microbial balance and cause digestive problems.

Vegetable oils: Soybean oil, maize oil, and canola oil are strong in omega-6 fatty acids, which may cause gastrointestinal inflammation.

Artificial Additives: Many processed meals include artificial colors, flavors, and preservatives, which may irritate the digestive system and cause gastrointestinal discomfort.

Excessive alcohol use may affect gut microbial balance, irritate the gut lining, and lead to diseases such as gastritis and acid reflux.

Processed Meats: Bacon, sausage, and deli meats often include nitrates and preservatives that may irritate the stomach and raise the risk of digestive problems.

rich-FODMAP Foods: Some fruits, vegetables, and sweeteners rich in fermentable carbs (FODMAPs) might aggravate symptoms of digestive disorders such as IBS and should be ingested in moderation.

CHAPTER TWO

Food Recipes For Digestive Health

Digestive health is essential for general well-being, and what we eat has a huge impact on sustaining it. Here is a comprehensive collection of 100 food dishes designed exclusively to promote digestive health, along with preparation instructions and amount measurements.

1. Overnight Oats

• Ingredients include rolled oats, yogurt, chia seeds, and fruit.

• Combine oats, yogurt, and chia seeds. Refrigerate overnight. Add the fruits just before serving.

2. Quinoa Salad

• Ingredients include quinoa, mixed veggies, olive oil, and lemon juice.

• To cook quinoa, use this procedure. Combine with chopped veggies. Drizzle with olive oil and lemon juice.

3. Baked Salmon

• Ingredients include salmon fillets, olive oil, lemon, and herbs.

• Marinate fish with olive oil, lemon, and herbs. Bake till tender.

4. Steamed vegetables

• Ingredients: Assorted veggies and spices.

• Procedure: Steam veggies until tender. Season to taste.

5. Miso Soup

• Ingredients include miso paste, tofu, seaweed, and green onions.

• Dissolve miso paste in boiling water. Combine tofu, seaweed, and green onions.

6. Whole Grain Toast

• Ingredients include whole grain bread, avocado, and tomatoes.

• Procedure: Toast bread. Spread avocado and top with cut tomatoes.

7. Lentil Soup

• Ingredients include lentils, carrots, celery, and vegetable broth.

• Cook lentils in vegetable broth with carrots and celery until tender.

8. Greek Yogurt Parfait.

• Ingredients include Greek yogurt, granola, berries, and honey.

• Procedure: Layer yogurt, granola, and berries. Drizzle with honey.

9. Brown rice

• Ingredients: Brown rice and water.

• Cook brown rice following package directions.

10. Spinach Salad

• Ingredients include spinach, strawberries, almonds, and balsamic dressing.

• Combine spinach, cut strawberries, almonds, and balsamic dressing.

11. Chicken and Vegetable Stir-Fry

• Ingredients include chicken breast, mixed veggies, and soy sauce.

• Stir-fry chicken and veggies in soy sauce until fully done.

12. Oat Bran Muffins

• Ingredients include oat bran, whole wheat flour, applesauce, and cinnamon.

• Procedure: Combine ingredients. Bake in a muffin tray until golden.

13. Poached eggs.

• Ingredients include eggs, water, and vinegar.

• To poach eggs, cook in boiling water with vinegar until set.

14. Sweet Potato Mash

• Ingredients include sweet potatoes, olive oil, and garlic.

• Method: Roast sweet potatoes. Mash in olive oil and garlic.

15. Tuna Salad

• Ingredients include canned tuna, Greek yogurt, celery, and onion.

• Combine tuna, Greek yogurt, chopped celery, and onion.

16. Whole grain pasta with vegetables

• Ingredients include whole-grain pasta, mixed veggies, and tomato sauce.

• Procedure: Cook pasta. Toss in the veggies and tomato sauce.

17. Baked Apples

• Ingredients include apples, cinnamon, and honey.

• Procedure: Core apples. Fill with cinnamon and honey. Bake till tender.

18. Vegetable Curry

• Ingredients include mixed veggies, curry paste, and coconut milk.

• Simmer veggies in curry paste with coconut milk until soft.

19. Chia Seed Pudding.

• Ingredients include chia seeds, almond milk, and vanilla essence.

• Procedure: Combine ingredients. Refrigerate until set.

20. Broccoli Soup

• Ingredients include broccoli, onion, garlic, and vegetable broth.

• Cook broccoli, onion, and garlic in vegetable broth. Blend until smooth.

21. Turkey Meatballs

• Ingredients include ground turkey, breadcrumbs, eggs, and seasonings.

• Procedure: Combine ingredients. Form into balls and bake until fully done.

22. Brown Rice Sushi Rolls

• Ingredients include brown rice, nori sheets, veggies, and avocado.

• Spread rice onto nori. Combine veggies and avocado. Roll tight.

23. Roasted Brussels sprouts.

• Ingredients include Brussels sprouts, olive oil, and balsamic vinegar.

• Toss sprouts with oil and vinegar. Roast till crisp.

24. Hummus and Vegetable Wraps

• Ingredients include whole grain wrappers, hummus, and other veggies.

• Spread hummus onto wraps. Add veggies. Roll and slice.

25. Chicken Bone Broth

• Ingredients include chicken bones, veggies, and water.

• Simmer bones and veggies in water for many hours. Strain.

26. Mixed Berry Smoothie

• Ingredients include mixed berries, spinach, Greek yogurt, and almond milk.

• Procedure: Combine all ingredients and blend until smooth.

27. Baked cod

• Ingredients include cod fillets, lemon, garlic, and herbs.

• Marinate fish with lemon, garlic, and herbs. Bake till flaky.

28. Quinoa Stuffed Peppers

• Ingredients include bell peppers, quinoa, black beans, and salsa.

• To cook quinoa, use this procedure. Combine with beans and salsa. Stuff the peppers and bake.

29. Cucumber Salad

• Ingredients include cucumber, tomatoes, red onion, and feta cheese.

• Combine chopped veggies with crumbled feta. Dress in olive oil.

30. Whole-Grain Pancakes

• Ingredients include whole grain flour, eggs, milk, and baking powder.

• Procedure: Combine ingredients. Cook on the griddle until browned.

31. Roasted Garlic Broccoli.

• Ingredients include broccoli, garlic, and olive oil.

• Toss broccoli with minced garlic and olive oil. Roast until tender.

32. Turkey Chili

• Ingredients include ground turkey, beans, tomatoes, and chili powder.

• Cook turkey, beans, tomatoes, and chili powder until flavors combine.

33. Almond Butter and Banana Toast

• Ingredients include whole-grain bread, almond butter, and bananas.

• Procedure: Toast bread. Spread with almond butter and top with sliced banana.

34. Vegetable frittata

• Ingredients: Eggs, various veggies, and cheese.

• Procedure: Beat eggs. Combine with veggies and cheese. Bake until completely set.

35. Baked sweet potatoes.

• Ingredients include sweet potatoes, olive oil, and rosemary.

• Procedure: Rub potatoes with oil and rosemary. Bake till tender.

36. Greek Salad

• Ingredients include cucumber, tomatoes, olives, and feta cheese.

• Toss the veggies with crumbled feta. Drizzle with olive oil and lemon juice.

37. Lentil Salad

• Ingredients include lentils, bell peppers, red onion, and parsley.

• Procedure: Cook lentils. Mix in the chopped veggies and herbs.

38. Banana Oatmeal Cookies

• Ingredients include bananas, oatmeal, honey, and cinnamon.

• Procedure: Mash bananas. Combine with oatmeal, honey, and cinnamon. Bake till golden.

39. Vegetable broth

• Ingredients: Mixed veggies, water, and herbs.

• Step: Simmer veggies and herbs in water. Strain.

40. Grilled Chicken Caesar Salad.

• Ingredients include grilled chicken breast, romaine lettuce, and Caesar dressing.

• Instructions: Grill chicken. Toss in lettuce and dressing.

41. Brown Rice Congee.

• Ingredients include brown rice, chicken broth, and ginger.

• Simmer rice and ginger in broth until porridge-like consistency.

42. Baked Zucchini

• Ingredients include zucchini, parmesan cheese, and breadcrumbs.

• Coat zucchini with Parmesan and breadcrumbs. Bake till crisp.

43. Black Bean Soup

• Ingredients include black beans, onion, garlic, and cumin.

• Cook beans with onion, garlic, and cumin until softened. Blend until smooth.

44. Tofu Stir-Fry

• Ingredients include tofu, mixed veggies, and soy sauce.

• Stir-fry tofu and veggies with soy sauce until well cooked.

45. Berry Chia Jam

• Ingredients include berries, chia seeds, and honey.

• Cook berries until softened. Mash with chia seeds and honey.

46. Vegetable and Bean Burritos

• Ingredients include whole grain tortillas, mixcd veggies, and beans.

• Fill tortillas with veggies and beans. Roll and bake till crispy.

47. Lemon Garlic Shrimp

• Ingredients include shrimp, lemon, garlic, and olive oil.

• Marinate shrimp with lemon, garlic, and olive oil. Grill till pink.

48. Buckwheat pancakes.

• Ingredients include buckwheat flour, eggs, milk, and baking soda.

• Procedure: Combine ingredients. Cook on the griddle until browned.

49. Roasted Beet Salad.

• Ingredients include beets, goat cheese, walnuts, and balsamic glaze.

• Procedure: Roast beets. Toss in goat cheese and walnuts. Drizzle with a balsamic glaze.

50. Vegetarian Omelette

• Ingredients include eggs, mixed veggies, and cheese.

• Procedure: Beat eggs. Cook with the veggies and cheese until done.

51. Chia Seeds Smoothie Bowl

• Ingredients include chia seeds, almond milk, bananas, and toppings.

• Blend chia seeds, milk, and bananas. Top with any preferred toppings.

52. Baked chicken breasts.

• Ingredients include chicken breasts, herbs, and olive oil.

• Marinate the chicken in herbs and oil. Bake until fully done.

53. Cabbage Salad

• Ingredients include shredded cabbage, carrots, and apple cider vinegar.

• Mix cabbage and carrots with vinegar. Allow to marinate before serving.

54. Turkey and Vegetable Skewers

• Ingredients include turkey breast, bell peppers, onions, and marinade.

• Procedure: Thread turkey and veggies on skewers. Grill until cooked.

55. Buckwheat Porridge

• Ingredients include buckwheat groats, milk, and honey.

• Instructions: Cook buckwheat with milk until tender. Sweeten with honey.

56. Tomato Basil Soup

• Ingredients include tomatoes, basil, onion, and garlic.

• Cook tomatoes, onion, and garlic until softened. Combine with basil.

57. Eggplant Parmesan

• Ingredients include eggplant, breadcrumbs, and marinara sauce.

• Coat eggplant slices with breadcrumbs. Bake in marinara sauce until tender.

58. Cucumber Gazpacho.

• Ingredients include cucumbers, tomatoes, bell peppers, and olive oil.

• Combine cucumbers, tomatoes, and peppers with olive oil until smooth. Chill before serving.

59. Turkey and Kale Stuffed Peppers

• Ingredients include ground turkey, kale, quinoa, and seasonings.

• Instructions: Cook turkey with greens and quinoa. Stuff the peppers and bake.

60. Chia Seed Lemonade

• Ingredients include chia seeds, lemon juice, honey, and water.

• Combine chia seeds, lemon juice, honey, and water. Allow to settle until gel-like.

61. Roasted Carrot Soup

• Ingredients include carrots, ginger, and coconut milk.

• Method: Roast carrots with ginger. Blend in coconut milk until smooth.

62. Grilled Vegetable Skewers.

• Ingredients: Assorted veggies and marinade.

• Marinate veggies. Grill until tender and faintly browned.

63. Avocado & Tomato Salad

• Ingredients include avocado, tomatoes, red onion, and cilantro.

• Toss sliced avocado, tomatoes, onion, and cilantro. Dress with lime juice.

64. Turkey and Quinoa Stuffed Mushrooms

• Ingredients include mushrooms, ground turkey, quinoa, and herbs.

• Stuff mushrooms with a turkey-quinoa combination. Bake until the mushrooms are soft.

65. Banana Walnut Bread

• Ingredients include bananas, whole wheat flour, walnuts, and honey.

• Procedure: Combine ingredients. Bake until golden and cook thoroughly.

66. Brussels Sprout Salad

• Ingredients include shredded Brussels sprouts, almonds, and cranberries.

• Toss Brussels sprouts, almonds, and cranberries. Dress with vinaigrette.

67. Sautéed spinach.

• Ingredients include spinach, garlic, and olive oil.

• Sauté spinach and minced garlic until wilted. Drizzle with olive oil.

68. Lentils and Vegetable Curry

• Ingredients include lentils, mixed veggies, and curry sauce.

• Cook lentils and veggies in curry sauce until soft.

69. Baked acorn squash.

• Ingredients include acorn squash, maple syrup, and cinnamon.

• Halve the squash. Drizzle with syrup and season with cinnamon. Bake until soft.

70. Greek Yogurt with Berries Popsicles

• Ingredients include Greek yogurt, mixed berries, and honey.

• Combine yogurt, berries, and honey. Pour into popsicle molds and freeze.

71. Stuffed Bell Peppers

• Ingredients include bell peppers, quinoa, black beans, and salsa.

• To cook quinoa, use this procedure. Combine with beans and salsa. Stuff the peppers and bake.

72. Chia Seeds Breakfast Bowl

• Ingredients include chia seeds, almond milk, fruit, and almonds.

• Combine chia seeds and milk. Allow to sit until thickened. Top with fruits and nuts.

73. Grilled Lemon Herb Chicken

• Ingredients include chicken breast, lemon, herbs, and olive oil.

• Marinate the chicken with lemon, herbs, and oil. Grill till cooked through.

74. Mixed Vegetable Soup

• Ingredients: Mixed veggies, vegetable broth, and herbs.

• Procedure: Cook veggies in broth with herbs until soft.

75. Oat Bran Pancakes.

• Ingredients include oat bran, eggs, milk, and baking powder.

• Procedure: Combine ingredients. Cook on the griddle until browned.

76. Baked cod with lemon.

• Ingredients include cod fillets, lemon, garlic, and olive oil.

• Marinate fish with lemon, garlic, and oil. Bake till flaky.

77. Black Bean and Corn Salad

• Ingredients include black beans, maize, bell peppers, and lime juice.

• Procedure: Combine beans, corn, and peppers. Dress with lime juice.

78. Turkey and Vegetable Soup

• Ingredients include ground turkey, mixed veggies, and broth.

• Instructions: Cook turkey with veggies in broth until flavors combine.

79. Mashed Cauliflower

• Ingredients: Cauliflower, garlic, and butter.

• Procedure: Steam cauliflower. Mash in garlic and butter.

80. Tomato & Avocado Salsa

• Ingredients include tomatoes, avocado, onion, and cilantro.

• Dice the tomatoes, avocado, and onion. Combine with chopped cilantro.

81. Buckwheat noodles with stir-fried vegetables

• Ingredients include buckwheat noodles, mixed veggies, and soy sauce.

• Procedure: Cook noodles. Stir-fried with veggies and soy sauce.

82. Chicken & Rice Soup

• Ingredients include chicken breast, rice, carrots, and celery.

• Instructions: Cook chicken, rice, carrots, and celery in stock until cooked.

83. Baked Pumpkin

• Ingredients include pumpkin, maple syrup, and cinnamon.

• Procedure: Slice the pumpkin. Drizzle with syrup and season with cinnamon. Bake until soft.

84. Quinoa Breakfast Bowl

• Ingredients include quinoa, almond milk, almonds, and fruits.

• To cook quinoa, use this procedure. Top with almond milk, almonds, and fruit.

85. Veggie and Tofu Stir-Fry

• Ingredients include tofu, mixed veggies, and soy sauce.

• Stir-fry tofu and veggies with soy sauce until well cooked.

86. Chickpea Salad

• Ingredients include chickpeas, cucumber, cherry tomatoes, and feta cheese.

• Combine chickpeas, chopped cucumber, tomatoes, and crumbled feta.

87. Apple Cinnamon Oatmeal

• Ingredients include rolled oats, apples, cinnamon, and honey.

• Cook oats with chopped apples, cinnamon, and honey until soft.

88. Roasted Cauliflower

• Ingredients include cauliflower, olive oil, and garlic powder.

• Toss cauliflower with oil and garlic powder. Roast until golden.

89. Spinach and mushroom quesadillas

• Ingredients include spinach, mushrooms, whole wheat tortillas, and cheese.

• Fill tortillas with sautéed spinach, mushrooms, and cheese. Grill until the cheese melts.

90. Lentil and Kale Salad

• Ingredients include lentils, kale, red onion, and feta cheese.

• Procedure: Cook lentils. Combine with chopped kale, onion, and crumbled feta.

91. Banana-Almond Smoothie

• Ingredients include bananas, almond milk, and almond butter.

• Process: Blend bananas, almond milk, and almond butter until smooth.

92. Grilled Vegetable Wrap.

• Ingredients include grilled veggies, healthy grain wraps, and hummus.

• Fill the wrap with grilled veggies and hummus. Roll and slice.

93. Baked Chicken Meatballs.

• Ingredients include ground chicken, breadcrumbs, eggs, and seasonings.

• Procedure: Combine ingredients. Form into balls and bake until fully done.

94. Quinoa & Black Bean Salad

• Ingredients include quinoa, black beans, bell peppers, and lime juice.

• To cook quinoa, use this procedure. Mix in the beans, peppers, and lime juice.

95. Green Smoothie

• Ingredients include spinach, kale, banana, and almond milk.

• Blend spinach, kale, banana, and almond milk until smooth.

96. Stuffed Acorn Squash

• Ingredients include acorn squash, quinoa, cranberries, and nuts.

• Instructions: Cook squash. Fill with cooked quinoa, cranberries, and walnuts.

97. Tomato Basil Quinoa

• Ingredients include quinoa, tomatoes, basil, and garlic.

• To cook quinoa, use this procedure. Toss in diced tomatoes, basil, and garlic.

98. Chickpea & Spinach Curry

• Ingredients include chickpeas, spinach, curry paste, and coconut milk.

• Cook chickpeas and spinach in curry paste and coconut milk until cooked through.

99. Apple Walnut Salad

• Ingredients include apples, walnuts, mixed greens, and balsamic vinaigrette.

• Combine sliced apples and walnuts with mixed greens. Dress with a balsamic vinaigrette.

100. Veggie and Brown Rice Stir-Fry

• Ingredients include mixed veggies, brown rice, and soy sauce.

• Stir-fry veggies, cooked brown rice, and soy sauce until heated through.

These 100 dishes provide a variety of possibilities for improving digestive health. Incorporating these healthy meals into your diet might help to enhance digestion and general health. Remember to pick a range of meals and consume them in moderation for the best effects.

CHAPTER THREE

The Function Of Fiber In Digestive Health

Fiber is important for digestive health because it promotes regular bowel movements, prevents constipation, and helps healthy bacteria proliferate in the stomach. Here's why it matters:

1. Promotes Regular Bowel Movements: Fiber bulks up stool, making it easier to move through the digestive system. This helps to avoid constipation and improves regularity.

2. Prevents Constipation: Insoluble fiber, found in whole grains, nuts, and vegetables, bulks up stool and allows it to flow more rapidly through the intestines, so avoiding constipation.

3. Supports healthy Bacteria: Certain forms of fiber, known as prebiotics, feed healthy bacteria in the

stomach. Fiber helps intestinal health by feeding microbes.

4. Regulates Blood Sugar Levels: Soluble fiber, found in foods such as oats, beans, and fruits, delays sugar absorption, hence stabilizing blood sugar levels. This may help lower the risk of insulin resistance and type 2 diabetes.

5. Reduces Cholesterol: Soluble fiber attaches to cholesterol particles in the digestive system, preventing them from being absorbed into the circulation. This may help decrease LDL (bad) cholesterol levels, lowering the risk of heart disease.

6. Weight Management: High-fiber foods are frequently low in calories, making you feel full and pleased after meals. This may help with weight control by lowering total calorie consumption.

7. Fiber promotes colon health by lowering the risk of colorectal cancer and other digestive diseases including diverticulosis.

8. Fiber regulates the release of digestive hormones including ghrelin and leptin, which are involved in hunger control and fullness.

9. Improves Gut Motility: Eating enough fiber helps calm muscular contractions in the digestive system, which promotes appropriate gut motility and prevents disorders like irritable bowel syndrome (IBS).

10. Improves Nutrient Absorption: Fiber promotes good digestion and regular bowel movements, resulting in optimum nutrient absorption from the foods we consume, supporting overall health and well-being.

Gut Healing Supplements And Herbs

In addition to dietary fiber, several vitamins, and herbs may help to improve digestive health and promote gut healing. Here are five prominent choices:

1. Probiotics: These helpful bacteria supplements may help balance the gut microbiota, improve digestion, and boost the immune system.

2. Digestive Enzymes: Supplementing with digestive enzymes may help with nutritional breakdown and absorption, particularly for those with digestive enzyme deficiencies or illnesses such as pancreatic insufficiency.

3. L-Glutamine: This amino acid is renowned for its ability to repair the intestinal lining and promote overall gut health. It may assist in relieving symptoms of leaky gut syndrome and inflammatory bowel illnesses.

4. Deglycyrrhizinated licorice (DGL) is a popular remedy for soothing and protecting the gastrointestinal system, especially in instances of gastritis, ulcers, and acid reflux.

5. Marshmallow Root: This plant includes mucilage, a gel-like material that coats and calms the digestive

system, making it effective in treating heartburn, indigestion, and inflammatory bowel illnesses.

6. Turmeric, with its powerful anti-inflammatory effects, may help decrease inflammation in the stomach and improve symptoms of illnesses such as ulcerative colitis and Crohn's disease.

7. Slippery Elm: Like marshmallow root, slippery elm contains mucilage, which coats and calms the digestive system, offering treatment for illnesses such as gastritis, GERD, and IBS.

8. Peppermint oil capsules may help ease symptoms of irritable bowel syndrome (IBS), such as stomach discomfort, bloating, and gas, by relaxing the muscles in the digestive system.

9. Ginger: Ginger is known for its digestive properties and may help relieve nausea, gas, and bloating, making it an effective herb for supporting overall gut health.

10. Aloe vera gel has anti-inflammatory and therapeutic characteristics that help calm and mend the intestinal lining, making it useful for ulcerative colitis and leaky gut syndrome.

The Gut Microbiome: Vital To Digestive Health

The gut microbiome, which includes billions of bacteria, fungi, and other microorganisms, is crucial to digestive health and general well-being. Understanding its relevance is critical for maintaining good gut function.

1. Microbial Diversity: A varied microbiome is linked to improved digestion, immunological function, and metabolic health. A diversified diet rich in fiber and fermented foods may help to increase microbial diversity.

2. Digestive Efficiency: Gut microorganisms help break down and ferment dietary fibers and other complex carbohydrates, generating short-chain fatty

acids (SCFAs) that feed the colon's cells and support gut health.

3. Immune Regulation: The gut microbiota works closely with the immune system, educating and regulating immune responses. A healthy microbiota may reduce inflammation and protect against autoimmune disorders.

4.   Neurotransmitter   Production: Gut microorganisms create neurotransmitters such as serotonin and dopamine, which are essential for mood management and mental wellness. An unbalanced microbiota has been associated with mood disorders such as sadness and anxiety.

5. Metabolic Health: Abnormalities in the gut microbiota have been linked to metabolic illnesses such as obesity, insulin resistance, and type 2 diabetes. Certain bacteria affect energy metabolism and fat storage.

6. Barrier Function: The gut microbiota serves to keep the intestinal barrier intact, preventing hazardous compounds from entering the circulation. Disruptions in this barrier function may result in diseases such as leaky gut syndrome.

7. Inflammation Regulation: Dysbiosis, or microbial imbalance, may cause chronic inflammation in the gut, leading to the development of inflammatory bowel illnesses (IBD) such as Crohn's disease and ulcerative colitis.

8. Vitamin Synthesis: Some gut bacteria can synthesize vitamins such as B vitamins and vitamin K, which are required for many metabolic activities in the body. A healthy microbiota promotes proper vitamin synthesis.

9. Antimicrobial Defense: helpful microbes in the gut create antimicrobial chemicals that help guard against pathogenic bacteria and illnesses, ensuring a

healthy balance of helpful and dangerous microorganisms.

10. Dietary Influence: Diet significantly influences the makeup and function of the gut microbiome. A diet high in fiber, fermented foods, and plant-based foods fosters a diversified and resilient microbiome.

CHAPTER FOUR

10-Day Meal Plan For Digestive Health

A well-planned diet may improve digestive health by supplying vital nutrients, encouraging regularity, and maintaining a healthy gut microbiota. Here's an example 10-day food plan created with digestive health in mind:

Day 1:

• Breakfast: overnight oats with mixed berries and chia seeds.

• Lunch: Quinoa salad with mixed veggies and grilled chicken.

• Dinner: Baked salmon with steamed broccoli and sweet potatoes.

Day 2:

• Breakfast includes whole grain toast with avocado and poached eggs.

• Lunch includes lentil soup with spinach and healthy grain bread.

• Dinner: Stir-fried tofu, bok choy, and brown rice.

Day 3:

• Breakfast: Greek yogurt, honey, and sliced almonds.

• Lunch: Chickpea salad with tomatoes, cucumbers, and feta cheese.

• Dinner: Grilled shrimp skewers with roasted veggies and quinoa.

Day 4:

• Breakfast: Smoothie with spinach, banana, almond milk, and protein powder.

• Lunch: Turkey and avocado wrap on whole grain tortilla.

• Dinner: Vegetable curry with tofu and brown rice.

Day 5:

• Breakfast: Whole grain cereal, almond milk, and sliced strawberries.

• Lunch: Spinach and feta-filled bell peppers.

• Dinner was grilled chicken breast with roasted Brussels sprouts and mashed cauliflower.

Day 6:

• Breakfast: Chia seed pudding with mango and shredded coconut.

• Lunch is quinoa tabbouleh with cucumber, tomato, and parsley.

• Dinner: Baked cod, steaming asparagus, and wild rice.

Day 7:

• Breakfast: Whole grain waffles topped with Greek yogurt and mixed berries.

• Lunch: black bean and corn salad with lime vinaigrette.

• Dinner is turkey meatballs with zucchini noodles and marinara sauce.

Day 8:

• Breakfast: omelet with spinach, mushrooms, and feta cheese.

• Lunch option: Roasted veggie and hummus wrap with healthy grain tortilla.

• Dinner: Grilled steak with roasted sweet potatoes and green beans.

Day 9:

• Breakfast: Protein pancakes with sliced banana and almond butter.

• Lunch: Quinoa and black bean stuffed peppers.

• Dinner: Baked chicken thighs served with roasted root veggies and quinoa.

Day 10:

• Breakfast includes avocado toast with cherry tomatoes and feta cheese.

• Lunch is lentil and vegetable soup with healthy grain bread.

• Dinner: Stir-fried tofu, mixed veggies, and brown rice.

This plan's meals are balanced with fiber-rich foods, lean proteins, healthy fats, and colorful fruits and vegetables to support digestive health, promote regularity, and feed the gut microbiota. Furthermore, keeping hydrated by drinking enough water throughout the day is critical for proper digestive function.

Digestive Health and Nutritional Absorption

Digestive health is important for general health since it impacts the body's capacity to absorb key nutrients from the diet. A functional digestive system ensures that nutrients are properly absorbed, which is essential for many biological activities such as energy generation, tissue repair, and immune system function.

The digestive process starts in the mouth, where enzymes convert food particles into smaller molecules. It continues in the stomach and small intestine, where further processing and nutrient absorption take place. Finally, waste products pass via the big intestine.

Chronic stress may have a substantial influence on digestive health by changing the balance of gut flora, raising inflammation, and affecting digestion. Mindfulness, meditation, exercise, and deep breathing are all stress management practices that may help you relax and improve your digestion.

The gut-brain axis connects the gut to the brain. Stress may interrupt this connection, resulting in digestive issues including IBS and functional dyspepsia.

Exercise For Digestive Health

Regular physical exercise improves digestive health by stimulating bowel movements, reducing constipation, and increasing overall gut motility. Exercise also increases blood flow to the digestive organs, hence improving nutrition absorption and digestive function.

Aerobic activity, such as walking, running, cycling, and swimming, may aid with digestion by raising heart rate and metabolism.

Sleep And Digestive Health

Quality sleep is critical for digestive health because it helps the body repair and rebuild tissues, including those found in the digestive system. Poor sleep habits, such as inconsistent sleep patterns or sleep deprivation, may impair digestive function and lead to gastrointestinal diseases.

Circadian Rhythm: The body's internal clock, or circadian rhythm, controls a variety of physiological functions, including digestion. Disruptions to this cycle, such as shift work or jet lag, might harm gut health.

Hydration And Digestive Health

Proper hydration is vital for supporting good digestion because it softens stool, prevents constipation, and aids in the transportation of nutrients through the digestive system. Water also helps with the breakdown and absorption of food particles.

Water Intake: To keep hydrated, it is advised that you drink at least eight glasses every day. Individual water requirements may vary depending on age, weight, activity level, and climate.

Probiotics & Digestive Health

Probiotics are helpful microorganisms that may assist in balancing the gut microbiota and promote digestive health. These living microbes may be found in foods like yogurt, kefir, sauerkraut, and kimchi, as well as in supplements.

Probiotics provide many benefits, including helping to maintain a healthy balance of gut flora, improving digestion, strengthening the immune system, and reducing symptoms of digestive problems including bloating, gas, and diarrhea.

CHAPTER FIVE

Fermented Food And Digestive Health

Fermented foods include beneficial bacteria that may improve digestive health by encouraging the development of healthy bacteria in the stomach. Consuming fermented foods daily helps improve digestion, decrease inflammation, and increase nutrient absorption.

Fermented foods may include yogurt, kefir, kombucha, miso, tempeh, sauerkraut, and kimchi. Incorporating these items into your diet will help you maintain a healthy gut microbiota and enhance digestion.

Finally, keeping excellent gut health is critical for general well-being and vigor. By combining stress management strategies, regular exercise, appropriate sleep, correct hydration, probiotics, and fermented foods into your lifestyle, you may promote optimum digestion and nutrient absorption, resulting in superior long-term health results.

Here Are 20 Natural Remedies For Constipation

1. Increase Fiber Intake: Fiber-rich foods such as fruits, vegetables, whole grains, and legumes bulk up stool, promoting regular bowel movements.

2. Stay Hydrated: Drinking enough water softens stool, making it easier to travel through the digestive system and reducing constipation.

3. Prunes: Prunes are a natural laxative because of their high fiber and sorbitol content, which promotes intestinal regularity.

4. Flaxseeds: High in fiber and omega-3 fatty acids, flaxseeds may help with constipation by increasing bowel movements.

5. Magnesium supplements or magnesium-rich foods, such as nuts, seeds, and leafy greens, may

help relax intestinal muscles, allowing for easier bowel movements.

6. Probiotics: Eating probiotic-rich foods such as yogurt, kefir, and fermented vegetables helps to maintain a healthy balance of gut bacteria, which can aid digestion and relieve constipation.

7. Castor oil is a natural laxative that stimulates bowel movements and relieves constipation when taken orally.

8. Exercise: Regular physical activity improves digestion and stimulates bowel movements, lowering the risk of constipation.

9. Aloe vera juice contains natural laxative properties that can help relieve constipation by stimulating bowel movements.

10. Senna tea and supplements containing senna extract can help with constipation by stimulating bowel contractions.

11. Dandelion Tea: Dandelion tea works as a gentle laxative and diuretic, promoting bowel movements and treating constipation.

12. Dissolving Epsom salt in water and drinking it can help with constipation by drawing water into the intestines and stimulating bowel movements.

13. Consuming a tablespoon of olive oil on an empty stomach can lubricate the intestines and encourage bowel movements, thereby relieving constipation.

14. Molasses: Blackstrap molasses contains magnesium and other minerals that can soften stool and relieve constipation.

15. Psyllium Husk is a soluble fiber supplement that when combined with water, can help regulate bowel movements and relieve constipation.

16. Herbal Teas: Some herbal teas, such as peppermint, ginger, and chamomile, have natural digestive properties that can help with constipation.

17. Warm Lemon Water: Drinking warm lemon water in the morning can stimulate digestion and promote bowel movements, thereby relieving constipation.

18. Coconut water is hydrating and rich in electrolytes, which helps soften stool and relieve constipation.

19. Figs are high in fiber and natural sugars, making them excellent for relieving constipation by encouraging bowel movements.

20. Both prune juice and apple juice contain sorbitol, a natural sugar alcohol that works as a laxative and may aid with constipation.

20 Cooking Techniques For Digestive Health

1.   Steaming preserves nutrients and facilitates simpler digestion than frying or boiling.

2. Grilling: Enhances tastes without adding too much fat, making foods gentler on the digestive system.

3. Poaching preserves the natural aromas and textures of dishes while using little additional lipids.

4. Baking uses dry heat to cook meals, retaining nutrients and facilitating easy digestion.

5. Stir-frying is a quick-cooking technique that keeps nutrition while adding flavor with minimum additional oil.

6. Broiling, like grilling, enables excess fat to drain away, resulting in lighter, more readily digested foods.

7. Raw: Eating raw fruits and vegetables maintains their natural enzymes and fiber levels, which improve digestion.

8. Blending: Produces smooth textures that are simpler to digest, particularly for those with digestive problems.

9. Slow-cooked soups and stews break down ingredients, making them more digestible while conserving nutrients.

10. Fermentation: Fermented foods such as yogurt, kimchi, and sauerkraut contain probiotics, which improve gut health and digestion.

11. Mashing softens and breaks down meals, making them simpler to digest, particularly for those who have difficulty chewing.

12. Roasting: Improves taste while conserving nutrients, resulting in readily digested foods.

13. Simmering is a slow cooking procedure that tenderizes and makes things easier to digest.

14. Pressure cooking preserves nutrients while immediately tenderizing foods, making them simpler to digest.

15. Marinating: Tenderizes meats and adds taste without using too much fat, making digestion easier.

16. Sous Vide is a precise cooking process that preserves nutrients and natural tastes, resulting in readily digestible food.

17. Boiling softens meals and retains nutrients, making them simpler to digest, particularly for those with sensitive stomachs.

18. Sautéing is a quick cooking process that enriches tastes while using little additional fats, enabling simpler digestion.

19. Simmering in broth adds flavor and moisture to meals, making them more digestible while also giving extra nutrients from the broth.

20. Steeping extracts taste and nutrients from herbs and spices, resulting in readily digestible infusions and teas.

Balancing Gut Flora And Prebiotics

Prebiotics are non-digestible fibers that nourish beneficial bacteria in the stomach, creating a balanced gut flora. Prebiotic-rich foods include garlic, onions, leeks, bananas, asparagus, and oats. Including these items in your diet may help promote the development of good bacteria and enhance digestive health.

The Importance Of Digestive Enzymes

Digestive enzymes are proteins that assist food break down into smaller molecules so that it may be absorbed. Bloating, gas, and indigestion may be caused by insufficient digestive enzyme synthesis. Supplementing with digestive enzymes or eating enzyme-rich foods such as pineapple, papaya, and fermented foods might help with digestion and relieve digestive pain.

Mindful Eating And Digestive Health

Mindful eating entails paying attention to the feelings and cues of hunger and fullness while eating. Chewing food completely, eating slowly, and enjoying each mouthful might help digestion by enabling enzymes in saliva to start the process and delivering signals to the brain that control hunger and digestion.

Addressing Food Sensitivity And Allergies

Identifying and eliminating foods that cause sensitivities or allergies may help relieve digestive problems including bloating, diarrhea, and stomach discomfort. Gluten, dairy, soy, eggs, and nuts are among the most common food allergies. Keeping a food diary and consulting with a healthcare expert may help you identify trigger foods and create a specific diet plan.

CHAPTER SIX

Supporting Liver Health And Digestion

The liver plays an important role in digestion by generating bile, which helps emulsify lipids for absorption. Supporting liver health with a balanced diet rich in fruits, vegetables, lean meats, and healthy fats, as well as limiting alcohol use and avoiding processed foods, may promote better digestion and general well-being.

Healing The Leaky Gut Syndrome:

Leaky gut syndrome occurs when the intestinal lining is compromised, enabling toxins, germs, and undigested food particles to enter the circulation, causing inflammation and digestive problems. To cure leaky gut, identify and remove trigger foods, reduce stress, and include gut-healing foods and supplements like bone broth, collagen, glutamine, and probiotics to repair the intestinal lining and restore gut health.

Managing Acid Reflux And Heartburn Naturally

Acid reflux and heartburn are typical digestive problems that may be easily treated with natural therapies. These disorders develop when stomach acid leaks back into the esophagus, producing pain and inflammation. While medicine is often administered, natural therapies may provide comfort while minimizing the danger of adverse effects.

Eating smaller, more frequent meals throughout the day is an excellent natural treatment for acid reflux and heartburn. This avoids overeating and relieves pressure on the stomach, lowering the probability of acid reflux. Avoiding trigger foods including spicy meals, caffeine, and citrus fruits may also help relieve symptoms.

Diarrhea may be annoying and painful, but several natural therapies might help. Increasing fluid intake is critical to avoiding dehydration, particularly while having frequent bowel movements. Consuming probiotic-rich foods like yogurt and kefir may also help restore the balance of good bacteria in the stomach, hence alleviating diarrhea symptoms.

Furthermore, certain herbal teas, such as chamomile and peppermint, have anti-inflammatory effects that help relax the digestive system and relieve diarrhea. Furthermore, integrating bland items into your diet, such as bananas, rice, and bread, will help bind stool and minimize bowel motions.

Relieving Bloating And Gas

Poor digestion often causes bloating and gas, which may be both painful and unsightly. Natural treatments may assist in reducing these symptoms and enhance digestive function. Consuming ginger tea or incorporating raw ginger into meals might help with digestion and prevent bloating.

Furthermore, include probiotics in your diet via foods like sauerkraut and kimchi may help maintain a healthy balance of gut flora, minimizing bloating and gas. Furthermore, limiting carbonated drinks and eating meals slowly and carefully might help you avoid swallowing additional air, which causes bloating.

Improving Digestive Health With Lifestyle Changes

Making lifestyle adjustments may help to enhance digestive health and avoid digestive problems. Regular exercise helps good digestion by increasing bowel movements and decreasing constipation. Furthermore, stress management practices such as meditation and deep breathing exercises might help avoid digestive issues including acid reflux and irritable bowel syndrome.

Furthermore, keeping hydrated by drinking enough water throughout the day promotes good digestion and avoids constipation. Furthermore, obtaining enough sleep each night is critical for digestive health, since inadequate sleep may disrupt digestion and increase symptoms of digestive diseases.

Developing A Support System For Digestive Health

Creating a support system is critical for sustaining digestive health, particularly when following a specific diet or coping with digestive problems. Being surrounded by supportive friends and family members may give encouragement and inspiration to keep to food restrictions and lifestyle adjustments.

Furthermore, joining online support groups or visiting local meetings for others dealing with similar digestive disorders may provide helpful information and support from those who understand what you're going through. Working with a healthcare expert, such as a nutritionist or gastroenterologist, may also give specific direction and assistance for successfully treating digestive difficulties.

CHAPTER SEVEN

The Gut-Brain Connection

The gut-brain connection refers to bidirectional communication between the gut and the brain, which is critical for digestive health and general well-being. Stress and worry may have a detrimental influence on digestion by disturbing gut bacterial balance and promoting inflammation.

Stress-reduction strategies like mindfulness meditation, yoga, and deep breathing exercises may assist improve digestive health by relaxing the nervous system and lowering gut inflammation. Furthermore, a diet high in fiber, fruits, and vegetables feeds the gut bacteria, encouraging a healthy gut-brain axis.

Dining Out On The Paleo Diet For Digestive Health

Following the Paleo diet when dining out might be difficult, but it is possible with proper planning and preparation. When eating out, choose places that provide Paleo-friendly dishes like grilled meats, fish, and salads with olive oil-based dressings.

Additionally, don't be afraid to question the restaurant staff about ingredient replacements or adjustments to meet your dietary requirements. Avoiding processed foods, wheat, and dairy products is essential for adhering to the Paleo diet when eating out and preserving intestinal health.

Traveling With The Paleo Diet For Digestive Health

Traveling while on the Paleo diet requires some additional preparation to ensure you have access to appropriate food selections. Before you go, look for restaurants and grocery shops in your region that provide Paleo-friendly foods including fresh fruits, veggies, and protein sources.

Additionally, try carrying portable Paleo snacks such as nuts, seeds, and dried fruit to have on hand when traveling. Additionally, having a small cooler with perishable Paleo-friendly meals will guarantee you have healthful alternatives accessible even while you're on the road.

Celebrate Holidays And Special Occasions On The Paleo Diet

Celebrating holidays and special events while on the Paleo diet may need some imagination, but it is feasible to enjoy great Paleo-friendly meals and desserts. When attending or hosting celebrations, provide Paleo-friendly foods that everyone may enjoy, such as roasted vegetables, grilled meats, and fruit salads.

Furthermore, explore creating Paleo-friendly adaptations of typical Christmas meals by substituting almond flour, coconut milk, and honey for grains, dairy, and processed sweets. Focus on the social parts of the celebration rather than just the food, and enjoy spending time with loved ones.

Overcoming Challenges And Setbacks

Despite best efforts, problems and setbacks are unavoidable whether dealing with digestive disorders or adhering to a certain diet, such as Paleo. It is critical to face setbacks with fortitude and a positive attitude, seeing them as chances for development and learning.

When experiencing a hardship, seek help from friends, family, or healthcare experts who may provide advice and encouragement. Furthermore, reassess your objectives and methods, making changes as required to overcome hurdles and remain on track in your gut health journey.

Tracking Progress And Symptoms

Tracking progress and monitoring symptoms is critical for properly treating digestive disorders and assessing the effectiveness of dietary and lifestyle modifications. Keep a food journal to track your meals, snacks, and any post-meal symptoms like bloating, gas, or diarrhea.

In addition, utilize symptom monitoring apps or notebooks to document changes in digestive problems over time and uncover trends or causes. Share this information with your healthcare provider to obtain tailored advice and changes to your treatment plan.

Maintaining Motivation On The Paleo Diet For Digestive Health

Staying motivated to follow the Paleo diet for digestive health requires commitment and devotion, particularly when confronted with hurdles or temptations. Remind yourself of the advantages of a healthy digestive system, including increased energy, mood, and general well-being.

Find inspiration by creating attainable objectives and appreciating tiny triumphs along the way. Surround yourself with people who support your health objectives and can provide encouragement and accountability. In addition, concentrate on the Paleo diet's tasty and healthy foods, experimenting with new dishes and tastes to make meals interesting and gratifying.

Conclusion

Managing digestive health naturally entails making lifestyle adjustments, dietary changes, and holistic techniques to relieve symptoms and increase overall well-being. Individuals who follow a Paleo diet, include natural therapies, and establish a strong support system may successfully manage digestive difficulties and enhance their quality of life.

Remember to remain motivated, measure your progress, and seek help when necessary to reach your long-term digestive health objectives.

9 798326 525635